SLIM GEMS: 10 PRICELESS WEIGHT LOSS

TECHNIQUES

by Matt Decker

I0419765

Published by THE DECKER EDGE

SLIM GEMS: 10 PRICELESS WEIGHT LOSS TECHNIQUES

GO TO THE GEM

INTRODUCTION

I know what it's like to fight the proverbial battle of the bulge. I know what it's like to struggle with weight. I have been engaged in that conflict since my childhood.

I have enduring memories of feeling bad about myself due to my weight, even eschewing short-sleeved shirts in order to cover the stretch marks on my arms. I can still recall the hurtful experiences of being labeled "fatboy," the comparison to the Pillsbury Doughboy and feeling that I was an inferior person because of my weight.

Happily, I also know what it's like to emerge victorious from this battle.

Beginning in 2007, I embarked on a weight loss journey which would lead to the shedding of more than 70 pounds of excess weight. Although I had lost a little weight at various points in the past, my victory dwarfed the successes of those previous attempts.

In a very real sense, I experienced a transformation - not only in terms of my appearance but also from a mental and emotional standpoint. For the first time in my life I achieved a feeling of self-confidence and positive self-esteem. I started to actually feel good about myself. It had less to do with the reduction in body fat and more to do with the knowledge that I had succeeded in transforming into a better version of myself. That was the goal, I achieved it and boy did it feel good.

I have been asked on multiple occasions how I managed to achieve such weight loss success. The question would usually be accompanied by a remark about the dramatic change in my appearance. Due to such questions I conceived the idea of sharing my story and disseminating the principles which I utilized to lose weight and gain health. Although the idea remained simmering in the back of my mind, I wasn't exactly sure how I could make it a reality. This book is the realization of that idea.

I adopted the ideas found in the following pages into my daily life. As a result, I succeeded in maintaining my improved health and fitness for five years. So I know they work when they are put to work.

Regrettably, I fell prey to depression and consequently abandoned the principles which brought me so much success. I am ashamed to admit that I allowed myself to gain every lost pound back. It didn't happen overnight. It was a gradual regression but that is usually how regression works.

But there is good news! I have rediscovered and returned to the ideas contained within these pages and am once again experiencing weight loss success. As of this writing, I have replicated my previous results to the tune of fifty-plus pounds.

GEM TIME

Gems are precious and beautiful. Gems are small. But despite their smallness, they are valuable. They have great worth. Gems permeate human language as a metaphor for something precious and valuable.

Why am I writing about gems in a book about weight loss? Consider this book a treasure chest of informational gems - valuable ideas - for empowering you to reach your health and fitness goals. I can attest to the value of these *Slim Gems* because I have experienced their sparkling brilliance in my own life. (Besides, the aforementioned term is also a clever wordplay on the famous beef snack, don't you think?)

As you make your way through the pages ahead, it's important to keep in mind that the ideas I write about are not theoretical. They are not untested and unproven theories. As stated above, I have put them to work in my own life and personally experienced their positive effects on my weight and my health.

As for *you*, dear reader - why not experiment with them yourself? Take them on a test drive of sorts. Try them out and watch what happens. I think you will be pleasantly surprised at the results.

Slim Gem #1: Straighten Up!

This technique is so simple, easy and straightforward that it's hard to believe it could make any real difference. But remember: things need not be complex and complicated in order to have a positive impact. *Gems are small but valuable.*

The simple practice of improving your posture won't literally take off any pounds, but it will make you appear that you have done so. This was the first Slim Gem I unearthed when I began my weight loss journey.

I got my hands on a little book titled *The Magic of Believing* by Claude Bristol, a self-help classic I would later learn. In the book, Bristol advocated the practice of a simple exercise which he dubbed "The Mirror Technique, " designed to improve self-confidence by tapping into the power of the subconscious mind. The exercise is no more complicated than standing up straight, while staring into the reflection of your eyes in the mirror. Since I didn't have an abundance of confidence in myself, I began to practice the technique with regularity.

I would stand in front of a mirror and practice straightening up my posture. I would even do it while sitting down. I did it so often that it became a habit. Every time I passed in front of a mirror my subconscious mind would prompt me to practice *posture training*. Not only did it instantly make me appear slimmer but it also improved my self-confidence and fueled my motivation.

I am in a special position to appreciate the value of proper posture (pardon the pun). Throughout my life, I have suffered from scoliosis which has curved my spine. The condition makes it even more important for me to attend to my posture.

And the idea behind this initial Slim Gem has been of considerable help. I know it will be of value to you as well.

The implementation of this idea is something you can do today. It doesn't require you to go without your favorite foods or break a sweat. It is a small but valuable daily practice which can help get you started on your weight loss journey.

Slim Gem #2: Diary Does Your Body Good

Feedback is an essential tool to improve any area of our lives. We can't fix what's wrong unless we know exactly where we are going wrong.

Think about a football team. The coaching staff uses the film of the previous week's game to show the players what they did wrong (and what they did right) on every play. What is the purpose of these film sessions? It is a form of feedback. We can take advantage of the same principle to improve our performance on the field of health and fitness.

What are we doing that is preventing us from reaching our goal weight? Where are we going wrong? The principle of feedback will help us answer those questions so we can make the necessary adjustments.

A simple (and inexpensive) way to provide ourselves with feedback for weight loss and weight management is to keep a detailed, written record of everything we eat and drink. This is known as a *food diary* or a *food journal.* The idea is as simple as writing down everything we eat and drink for a certain period of time (such as a week). It's also a good idea to record how we physically feel after eating specific foods.

The purpose of this particular Slim Gem is to gather raw data on our dietary patterns. Once we have that information, we can then make the necessary adjustments.

Furthermore, the very act of writing down what we are eating helps to get our impulses under control, regardless of the actual content of our observations. I know this because I have experienced the aforementioned positive effect on my own weight loss and weight management efforts.

An alternative idea to keeping a *written* food diary is to use your phone to *take photos* of what you eat and drink throughout the course of each day. This idea is more convenient for most people than writing the information down. Why? Because the average person today carries their phone around like it's an extra body part. It's a simple matter of whipping it out and snapping a pic of your food before eating it. Then you can review the pics at the end of the day to see where you can make some dietary corrections. After all, a picture is worth...well I think you know the rest.

On a personal note, I started out writing my eating patterns down on index cards. Then one day it occurred to me that I could achieve the same result without any written words by simply using my phone to take pics of my food. In fact, I think the picture method drove the points home even better than the written method.

Additionally, there are an assortment of food diary apps to choose from to help you utilize this concept even further. Computer scientists at Harvard University have even developed a crowdsourcing app that lets other Internet users analyze the photos you take of your food choices. (If you would like more information, google *PlateMate App*.)

Slim Gem #3: Look in Your Mental Mirror

In the classic fairy tale *Snow White*, the Evil Queen possesses a magic mirror - capable of answering her questions. Similarly, if you are struggling with your weight, it can seem that you possess a "talking" mirror of your own. Every time you step in front of it, that looking glass cruelly reminds you of your weight reality. It mocks you and spews discouragement at you.

The first Slim Gem pointed out the value of standing in front of a mirror to improve your posture. There is another type of mirror that you need to know about. This mirror is not made of glass and cannot be purchased at any home improvement store. But it is the nearest thing to a "magic mirror" in the real world. I am referring to your *mental mirror* - the mirror of your imagination.

16

You can experience the "magic" of this mirror via your imagination. Specifically, the idea is to create a mental image of the person you wish to become. In terms of weight loss, visualize the way you want to look. Visualize what you will look like after you have reached your goal weight. Project your thoughts to a point in time when your health and fitness goals have become a reality. Now imagine looking in a literal mirror. What image is staring back at you?

Psychology refers to this inner picture of ourselves as our *self-image.*

The year was 1960 and a book was published which would become a self-help classic, inspiring the teachings of future motivational giants such as Zig Ziglar and Tony Robbins. The book was titled *Psycho-Cybernetics*, authored by Maxwell Maltz. The core message of the book was that our self-image, be it positive or negative, works on a subconscious level to determine our success or failure. We cannot achieve success, Maltz wrote, as long as we hold a negative self-image. This concept applies to any and all areas of our lives, including of course our attempts at weight loss.

Maltz was a plastic surgeon before penning the wisdom of Psycho-Cybernetics. He wrote that his work as a plastic surgeon gave him an opportunity to witness the incredible power of the self-image to create either positive or negative results. Maltz noted the dramatic change in a patient's personality after undergoing a cosmetic procedure.

Conversely, he observed the phenomenon of a patient thinking nothing had changed with their appearance, despite a significant cosmetic difference having been performed. Maltz concluded that a person's mental picture of themselves functioned as a subconscious success (or failure) "mechanism".

"Our self image, strongly held, essentially determines what we become." ~Maxwell Maltz~

Good luck trying to become a slim person while "seeing" yourself as an overweight person. Good luck in reaching your goal weight while focusing on your present weight and identifying with that reality. Good luck because you will need luck. The point: in order to become the person you desire to be (which includes your desired level of health and fitness), it is necessary and essential for you to align your self-image (the mental picture you hold of yourself) with your desires.

You can't transform into a butterfly as long as you see yourself as a caterpillar.

"The Transformation Chamber"

Imagine that you have access to a magical transformation chamber or booth. Imagine stepping into your transformation chamber. Now imagine stepping out - transformed into the highest version of yourself.

What do you look like? How is your body different from your present body? Far more importantly, how do you feel? How is your attitude and personality different? This is a simple visualization technique which is designed to help you form a clear mental image of a leaner, fitter, healthier, better you. I know from experience that it works.

Slim Gem #4: Walk It Off!

When we are feeling angry or upset, we are often told to just "walk it off". The idea behind the advice is to walk until we are able to recover from the temporary emotional state which is causing us distress. It means to walk until we are able to shake the emotional monkey off our backs. The physical action of going for a walk gives us the opportunity to "blow off steam" in a healthy way.

Similarly, we can walk off the *physical baggage* known as excess weight by the daily habit of putting one foot in front of the other. This baggage didn't accumulate overnight and it won't disappear overnight. But we *can* walk it off if we are committed.

I know from whence I write. I walked off seventy-plus pounds. Sure, I did other things as well (hence the reason for this book) but the daily habit of walking was central to the dramatic improvement of my health and fitness.

Conversely, I can trace my regaining of weight to the ill-advised decision to stop walking everyday due to my fall into depression.

"Walking is man's best medicine." ~Hippocrates~

The man from whose mind the above quote originated knew a thing or two about medicine. Hippocrates was a Greek physician who lived before the time of Christ. He is considered the father of Western medicine. Every physician practicing today is well acquainted with the Hippocratic Oath. Although many centuries have passed since Hippocrates praised walking as the best medicine one could "take", modern science is confirming his ancient prescription. In fact, there is a steady stream of research spotlighting the enormous health benefits of simply putting on your walking shoes each day.

Walking is indeed nature's "medicine" for a host of ills and ailments, including the daily struggle to attain higher levels of health and fitness. You really can *walk it off*!

Slim Gem #5: Mind Control = Portion Control

Portion control is essential to weight loss and weight management. Perhaps you have noticed how portion sizes have gotten out of control in our society, particularly within the American diet and food industry. We live in a world of super-sized fast food meals, Big Macs, Big Gulps and jumbo-sized movie theater popcorn. The expansion of our food portions has occurred parallel to the expansion of our waistlines. Could this *really* be a mere coincidence? The magnitude of this "portion distortion" is so great that it is forcing the marketplace to respond with downsized products.

The good news: there are very simple techniques you can use to trick your brain (and belly) into exercising portion control and becoming satisfied with far less. Mind control really does equal portion control because it is all regulated by what's going on in your head.

One very simple idea is to *make a fist* before eating anything. How could something as simple as making a fist possibly help you control your portions and thus help you control your weight? The act of making a fist serves as a reminder - a visual cue - to your brain as to how big of a portion of food you should eat. As you look at your balled-up fist, you are instantly reminded to keep your portion of a particular food choice to that appropriate size. Don't let the simplicity of this idea fool you into thinking it can't work.

This next technique for portion control is quite powerful because it makes use of the most powerful form of human thought - namely, *visualization*. Before eating (or drinking) anything, take a few moments to visualize or imagine cutting the food in half, eating only fifty percent of it and saving the rest for later. Practice this visualization technique even if you don't think you have the willpower to only consume half of your food. That doesn't matter.

All you have to do is *imagine* cutting your food in half. That's it. Our brains cannot tell the difference between a real experience and one which is *vividly imagined*. If you visualize it enough, you will eventually find yourself physically doing it.

I know this idea works because I have experimented with it and experienced its amazing effect. If you mess up and neglect to do it before you eat, you can think about what you've already eaten and imagine *what if* you had cut it in half and only eaten fifty percent of it. If you give this idea a chance, I think you will be amazed at the results. I know I have been.

A third technique for portion control is to simply downsize the plates, bowls, cups and eating utensils you use for your meals and snacks. Use smaller versions of the kitchenware you are using now.

Research has shown that, if you have a large portion of food before you, then you will eat accordingly. The solution is to have smaller portions before you. You can do this by simply eating and drinking from smaller plates, bowls, glasses, etc. It is a very simple method for tricking your brain into consuming less, and that is the essence of portion control.

Slim Gem #6: Focus on the Right Number

Too often we get hung up on that depressing number we see displayed on the bathroom scale. It's like a neon sign reminding us of how far we are from our goal weight.

The solution is to shift our focus from that number to another, more positive number: the number we *will* see on that glorious day when we have reached our desired weight. Focus on that future number.

THE POWER OF F.O.C.U.S.

A good way to think about the power and meaning of focus is to convert the word itself into an acronym. What is focus? It is the *(f)aculty (o)f (c)reating (u)nder (s)tress.*

There is very real stress attached to your present weight - especially when it is so far from where you want to be. Nevertheless, you can successfully create positive results - despite the stress - by focusing on your goal weight. Focus is a faculty, and a powerful one at that. Use it.

Keep in mind that the number you see right now is only temporary. It will change, it will go down, as you take each step toward your health and fitness goal.

A simple way to get your focus in a better place is to write down the number of your goal weight. Mentally project yourself to the future date when you have won your personal battle of the bulge. When you step on the scale on that future date and a big smile comes across your face, what do you see when you look down? The answer is your goal weight. Write *that* number down and focus on it.

There are two ways to "cash in" this particular Slim Gem. You can either write it down every day or you can write it once and post it in a place where you will see it often. Why not stick it on your bathroom scale (or at least *near* your bathroom scale)? This simple idea will help you focus on the positive goal in your future rather than getting stuck in the frustration of your present weight.

Slim Gem #7: Think Like a Vegan

» Study: Vegan Diets Healthier For Planet, People Than Meat Diets

» Vegan Buddhist Nuns Have Same Bone Density As Non-vegetarians

» Vegetarian diets associated with lower risk of death

» Low-carb vegan diet may reduce heart disease risk, weight

» Vegan diet best for weight loss even with carbohydrate consumption, study finds

» To shed weight, go vegan

The above news headlines were born from the results of scientific studies spanning nearly a decade. No one "in the know" would quibble with the notion of the health value of a vegan diet

31

(meaning an animal-free, plant-based diet). In fact, it's more than a notion. As the above headlines attest, it is science.

I appreciate the fact that many people consider the idea of going vegan to be extreme and not something they think they could ever stick to. My goal here is not to persuade anyone to take that major dietary leap. However, you don't have to become a vegan in order to start *thinking* like a vegan.

You can think like a vegan by focusing on making fruits and vegetables the main component of your diet. You can think like a vegan by making a conscious effort to eat fruits and vegetables everyday instead of unhealthy, fattening processed food. You can begin to think like a vegan by asking yourself, before putting anything in your body, "Did this come from nature?".

Be careful, though. If you start thinking like a vegan, you may very well become one. It could result in better health and a smaller waistline. But there are worst things, right?

Slim Gem #8: Make the Switch

Most of us associate dieting and weight loss in general with pain. We associate the process with deprivation and there is nothing fun about deprivation (unless you live in a monastery).

This negative association is most unfortunate because it is not grounded in truth. *The battle of the bulge is won, not by deprivation, but by switching to healthier alternatives and choosing better options.*

Again we are led back to the power of focus. We must shift our focus from what we can no longer have to all the new, healthier, better things we *can* have and enjoy.

I lost five pounds without changing anything I was eating by simply applying this principle.

I was drinking a lot of sugary sodas. I sat down with a calculator and added up all the calories I was putting into my body solely from the soda. The total was more than 700 calories per day - just from what I was drinking! My food intake didn't even factor into the total.

It occurred to me, with the aforementioned principle of alternatives in mind, that I could achieve a dramatic reduction in my daily caloric consumption simply by *switching* to a diet beverage which suited my taste - without even making any alteration to my food intake. I figured that such a switch *had* to result in weight loss. I was correct - I lost five pounds by that single, painless idea.

For many years I was tormented by a skin condition on my hands. I suffered from incessant itching and my hands would break out in a terrible rash. It got to the point where I would wear gloves in public (regardless of the weather) because my hands were in such terrible shape. I could find no relief.

I tried everything I could think of. I went to multiple doctors through the years but each one was baffled by the cause of my condition. They would prescribe me medication in the form of hand ointment and pills which I was grateful for. At least it blessed me with temporary relief. But it was no cure because the torturous condition would always return once the medication ran out.

To make a long story shorter, I finally had my "Eureka!" moment. It started out as a theory. I theorized that the source of my dermatological torment was an allergic reaction to commercial hand soaps. I decided to test the theory.

I was proven to be correct. I stopped using chemical-laden commercial hand soaps and started using an all-natural alternative in its place. The result: healing for my hands which had eluded me for so many years.

What does the above story have to do with losing weight? Although it's not directly connected, it illustrates the wonderful results which can be achieved by making healthy switches - whether the goal is healing for a skin condition or the burning of body fat.

Slim Gem #9: Your Week Point

If you are succumbing to weight gain, there is a strong possibility that you have *at least* one weak point. And it is equally likely that this weak point is habitually getting the upper hand. There is a solution.

*Turn your **weak point** into a **week point**.*

Take time on Sunday to target one fattening food in your diet. Set a goal to eliminate this weak point in your diet in the week ahead. Repeat this process with a new dietary target every Sunday. By employing this technique you can turn your weak point - be it cake, pizza or whatever - into your week point of focus.

It's amazing what can be accomplished within seven days. There are 168 hours in a given week. Each one of these hours can either make you fatter, make you slimmer or keep you in the same condition. The choice is yours as to how you use them. The slimmest person in the world doesn't have any extra hours or days. Think about it.

If you are consistent with this strategy, you will eventually remove every "fat-maker" from your weekly diet and thus your life.

Slim Gem #10: "Mixercise"

In a previous Slim Gem I shared how the daily habit of walking empowered me to dramatically improve my health and fitness. Once that simple habit was firmly planted in my daily routine I decided it was time to "kick it up a notch." I decided it was time to take my exercise routine (and thus my fitness) to a higher level.

I was able to accomplish this with an idea I like to call *mixercise*. It is more commonly known as interval training. I *mixed* or interspersed brief periods of jogging with my walking. I would walk as usual but every ten minutes or so I would jog for a short period, then return to my walking. I repeated this pattern throughout the time I had set aside to exercise.

This idea of *mixercise* (interval training) had the desired effect. It enabled me to burn more fat and get more from my walking.

There is no shortage of research findings and scientific studies concerning this concept of mixing brief, high-intensity bursts of exercise such as jogging with lower-intensity exercise such as walking. Mix it to fix it...your health and fitness, that is.

Of course you should consult with your physician before embarking on any exercise program, especially one that incorporates high-intensity components no matter how brief the intervals.

FAT-TO-FIT

Think about the words *fat* and *fit* - two seemingly opposite ends of the health spectrum. They are not, however, very far apart. In fact, the only thing that separates them is a single letter.

You can go from "fat" to "fit" by merely changing the *a* to an *i*. You can transform the negative into a positive by one simple switch - one vowel into another. Likewise, it doesn't require an enormous shift to transition from being overweight to being slim and (most important) healthy. Amazing results can be achieved by making simple changes. That's what this book has been about.

Gems are small but valuable.

Best wishes to you on your weight loss journey. I did it...so can you!

Other Books by Matt Decker

» Grace in a Maze: How to Make it Through

» Super Scriptures on Earth

Booklets

» Truth, Jesus and The Bible Way

» The Real Transformers

<All titles are available exclusively @

Amazon.com>